NASAL ALLERGY
TREATMENT ROADMAP

BENOIT D. TANO, MD, PhD

CONTENTS

Warning And Disclaimer

Integrative Medical Press has designed this book to provide information about Nasal Allergy Treatment Roadmap to help patients take better care of their nasal allergies. This information is derived from the author's practice of Allergy and Clinical Immunology and Integrative Immunity and is not intended to replace your physician. The publisher and the author are not liable for the misconception or misuse of the information provided in this book.

Every effort has been made to ensure that the information contained in this book is complete and accurate. The author and publisher assume neither liability nor responsibility to any person or entity with respect to any direct or indirect loss or damage caused, or alleged to be caused by the information contained herein, or for errors, omissions, inaccuracies or any other inconsistency within these pages.

INTRODUCTION

I am an allergist, clinical immunologist, author and public speaker dedicated to helping patients who are suffering from nasal allergies, allergic conjunctivitis (allergy-related eye symptoms), adult-onset allergies, eczema, asthma, food allergies, urticaria (hives)/angioedema (body swelling: face, lips, tongue, whole body), obesity, diabetes, hypertension, hyperlipidemia, hormone-related disorders and many other conditions. I am passionate about helping not only treat patients, but also about spreading the word about the causes and how to avoid them.

I am also passionate about teaching people how to avoid these conditions and about the lifestyle choices to make through seminars, public speaking and my books, *The Allergy Detective* and *Hormone Imbalance Syndrome*. Don't suffer through your condition unnecessarily; there is a treatment plan for you. I have designed a one-page treatment plan for some of the conditions mentioned above that I call the Treatment Roadmap series. This book is about the Nasal Allergy Treatment Roadmap. It is the description of my one-page nasal allergy treatment roadmap that you can master in 15-30 minutes for better treatment of your nasal and eye symptoms.

Many people today are suffering increasingly from allergies and allergic disorders, and they are confused about why this is the case and worried that they don't know what to do to feel better. Do you or someone you know suffer from allergies? Have you struggled to find a treatment that really works and have been frustrated that your allergies are getting worse over the years? Then Nasal Allergy Treatment Roadmap is for you.

Nasal allergies fall under four major categories:

1. Allergic rhinitis (inflammation of the nasal membranes due to pollens, dust, dust mites, molds, pet dander, etc.)
2. Non-allergic rhinitis (inflammation of the nasal membranes due to chemicals like household cleaning agents, cigarette smoke, perfumes, flower scents, scented candles, air fresheners, petrochemicals, fumes, etc.)
3. Allergic conjunctivitis (inflammation of the eyes causing itchy, watery, puffy, swollen, red eyes)
4. Sinusitis (acute and chronic sinus infections)

The bulk of allergy cases are treated by primary care health care providers. Many patients also self-treat, and the multiple over-the-counter (OTC) antihistamines available to the public attest to that. However, many health care providers do not have a deep understanding of the pathophysiology of rhinitis symptoms. Also, many patients who self-medicate tend to use the weakest antihistamines and, often, the more dangerous medications that lead to rhinitis medicamentosa (rebound nasal congestion), such as Oxymetazoline (Afrin®). Others use nasal decongestants, such as Phenylephrine (Neo-Synephrine®), compounds and a combination of antihistamines and decongestants that can lead to high blood pressure. Understanding the mechanisms behind nasal symptoms and using an optimal combination of medications is necessary for effective treatment of nasal symptoms that are not benign.

Untreated or poorly treated allergic and non-allergic rhinitis can lead to chronic and recurrent sinus infections, sinus pressure, headaches, and even to asthma symptoms of chest tightness, shortness of breath, coughing, and wheezing. Postnasal drip, which is present in most allergy patients, is one of the most annoying, difficult to treat, and lingering rhinitis symptoms.

Healthcare professionals may also learn a brief pathophysiology of allergic and non-allergic rhinitis, as well as treatment protocols and techniques that will help their patients. In most cases of rhinitis, finding out the allergens by skin testing and desensitization by allergy vaccines leads to long-term relief, and qualified allergists will offer this service. If allergy sufferers are only interested in palliation (lessening) of their symptoms, they can often get good results by knowing what OTC medications work best and which ones to avoid. In this guide, you will learn about the medications that can give you relief and how to save yourself money and grief.

This guide, drawn from my own practice experience as an allergist, is intended to help all allergy sufferers take better control of their allergies. I have noticed that many healthcare professionals do not have the time to thoroughly educate their patients about the root cause of their allergies. Prescription medication and over-the-counter (OTC) medications are not used optimally because of lack of explanation of the medication's use and techniques that yield optimal results. This guide is a treatment plan that I teach all my patients when they come to clinic. It is a one-page synopsis of what allergies are, what is causing the reactions, and how to better treat allergy symptoms for optimal relief.

ILLUSTRATIVE TYPICAL NASAL ALLERGY CASE

Chief Complaint (CC): Most patients present with seasonal/perennial (year-round) allergic rhinitis (inflammation of the nose, hay fever), perennial non-allergic rhinitis (multiple chemical sensitivities), acute or chronic sinusitis (sinus infections) and mild intermittent, mild persistent, moderate persistent and severe asthma symptoms. This guide will only concentrate on the nasal symptoms.

HISTORY OF PRESENT ILLNESS (HPI)

You live in the Midwest (south, east, or west in the U.S. or any other place on Earth), and you came to our clinic with the above complaints. You told us that you have always had allergy symptoms that started in childhood. Your symptoms consist of sneezing, runny nose, stuffy nose, itchy, watery, sometimes red and puffy eyes, and fullness in the ears, postnasal drainage that leads to coughing without wheezing, chest tightness or shortness of breath. You also get about one-two sinus infections per year requiring antibiotic treatment. You reported that your allergy triggers are: pollens, dust, molds, animal dander (cat, dog, maybe cattle, horses, rabbits, guinea pig, gerbils, etc.), cigarette smoke,

5

perfumes, household cleaning agents, and petrochemicals (car exhaust and diesel fuel). Your symptoms are year-round but tend to get worse in the spring and fall. You use over-the counter (OTC) antihistamines, such as Claritin, Zyrtec, or Benadryl, or decongestants, such as Sudafed or Mucinex, occasionally that partially help. You have not tried any steroid nasal sprays or saline nasal washes, and you have recently seen your primary care physician who recommended Claritin and subsequently switched you to Singulair. However, these medications only partially help. You feel that your allergy symptoms are getting worse over time, and you now want to know why you have allergies and what the mechanism is behind these allergies. You are sick and tired of being sick all the time. Above all, you want to know how to get rid of these chronic nasal symptoms for good, and that is the reason for your clinic visit.

In your allergy profile, you indicated that you had eczema as a child that resolved early on, and you have no asthma or food allergies, medication allergies or insect sting allergies. You do not have any other medical conditions. Both your parents have allergies, and you have two siblings who also have allergies.

REVIEW OF YOUR BODY SYSTEMS

I went from head to toes and asked you specific questions in order to find out other symptoms you may have that we have not talked about in your HPI. Your review of systems is only significant for symptoms already described above.

Your physical examination showed allergy shiners (darkening around the eyes that many allergy patients have), an allergic salute sign (a crease across the nose that some allergy sufferers have), marked swelling of the inferior turbinates in both nostrils with non-purulent mucus noted in both nostrils. Your throat is moderately red, which has been caused by postnasal drip, and your ears are clear (without infection). The rest of your physical examination was normal.

After your physical examination, I recommended a skin test to find out what is causing your allergy symptoms. You have given me several clues during this process by telling me what you are experiencing every day (in your **HPI**) and also by my personal observations from your physical examination.

After your skin test, I showed you the Allergy Treatment ROadMAp (**ATROMA**®=you can use this acronym to mean without trauma, for example), and systematically, we covered the **W**hy, the **W**hat, and the **Ho**w (**WWHO**®=Read as **WHO**; in future series, I will talk about your **WWHO**® as the reason for your visit) to treat your allergies. This allergy roadmap has made a difference in many patients' lives, and patients even share the message with their friends and family to help them with their allergies. I started using this roadmap as an educational tool as soon as I started practicing allergy and immunology in 2006.

In 2008, while working for the U.S. Army in Northern Virginia, I drew the roadmap for one of my patients as I do for all the patients; this patient was so impressed with his results that he decided to send my scribbled roadmap to his wife who lived in Wisconsin at the time so that she could take the roadmap to her doctor for better treatment of her allergies. After that encouraging encounter, I decided to draw the roadmap on the computer. I have since used the computer version in all my patient education sessions and seminars. The roadmap is also published in my books *The Allergy Detective: Allergic Rhinitis Treatment Secrets Your Doctor May Not Tell You* and in The *Hormone Imbalance Syndrome: America's Silent Plague.* Since most patients report feeling well once they go through the **WWHO** technique, I have decided to share this one-page allergy treatment roadmap that I call the Nasal Allergy Treatment Roadmap with the rest of the world. You can find more detailed information and references in my books and you will find the Amazon link for these books at the end of this **ATROMA**.

I have come to realize that if you are suffering from allergies or any other illnesses, you have less time and patience to read several hundred-page books that may take you several hours or days before you know your **WWHO** for your illness. This book is conceived to be **short, concise and full of pearls** to help you treat your symptoms within **15-30 minutes**. Reading the whole book will take you about **30 minutes**. I will make available other treatment roadmaps that I use in my clinic in future books, so look out for those on my website www.drbtano.com.

The next page shows you the one-page diagram of my Nasal Allergy Treatment Roadmap. The rest of the pages describe step by step what is in this roadmap. If you follow the description of the roadmap, you will understand within 30 minutes why you have allergies, what immune cells are involved, and how you can successfully treat your nasal allergies by using existing OTC medications, prescription medications, and/or immunotherapy (**SCIT=subcutaneous immunotherapy** or allergy shots, and **SLIT=sublingual immunotherapy** or allergy drops) and where to find help for long-term relief.

NASAL ALLERGY TREATMENT ROADMAP

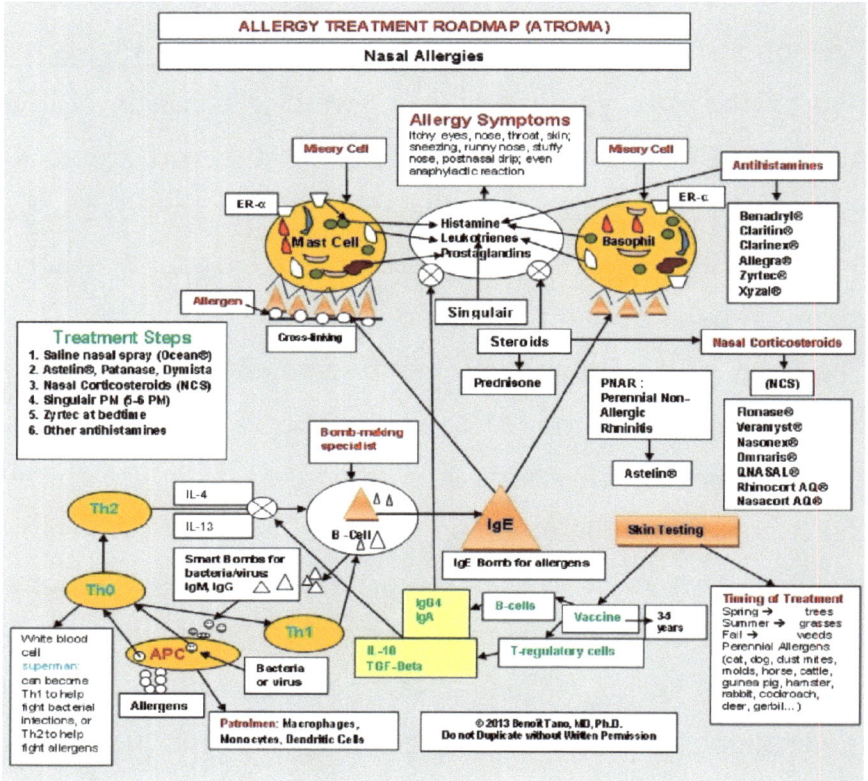

ALLERGY TREATMENT ROADMAP (ATROMA®)

WHY AM I HAVING NASAL ALLERGY SYMPTOMS?

Your first question for your clinic visit is, "Why do I have these allergy symptoms (and other people do not)?"

- ❖ For some individuals, allergies start in childhood.
- ❖ These individuals tend to inherit the genes from one or both of their parents.
- ❖ If one parent has allergies, the child has about a 40% chance of developing allergies.
- ❖ If both parents have allergies, the child has about a 70-90% chance of developing allergies.
- ❖ If neither parent has allergies, the child has about a 10 to 15% chance of developing allergies.
- ❖ The allergy gene alone does not cause allergic reactions.
- ❖ To react, the individual has to have the gene and be in the right environment.
- ❖ Gene-environmental interactions lead to allergic reactions.
- ❖ The prevalence of allergic diseases in the developed world is partially explained by the hygiene hypothesis, which holds that allergies are due to too much cleanliness.

❖ In developing countries, people's immune systems are busy fighting widespread bacteria, viruses, protozoa and parasites and have no time to concentrate on innocuous substances, such as pollens and other allergens.

❖ In the developed world where individuals are not exposed to bacteria as much, the immune system, looking for work, turns to fighting innocuous substances such as pollens. There are three diseases that go together and are known collectively as atopic diseases: atopic dermatitis (eczema), asthma, and allergic rhinitis (ear, nose and throat symptoms).

❖ There is something called the atopic march, which is a progression of atopic diseases in which children start with eczema around age four-five months, when they are first exposed to solid foods.

❖ By age three-four months, (sometimes sooner and other times later), some children develop upper respiratory infections, such as respiratory syncytial virus (RSV) infection and other viral infections that lead to their first wheeze, cough, shortness of breath and chest tightness (asthma symptoms).

❖ These symptoms, often called reactive airway disease by many primary care physicians, may continue until adulthood, or may subside early in childhood.

- By age two, most children with atopy have developed their allergic rhinitis symptoms.
- Sometimes, the sequence is eczema-allergic rhinitis-asthma, or asthma-eczema-allergic rhinitis.
- If the children develop allergic rhinitis that is untreated or poorly treated, they can develop asthma symptoms as a consequence; that is known as allergic rhinitis impact on asthma. Chronic sinusitis is a consequence of a poorly treated rhinitis. When mucus does not drain from the sinuses, it becomes a breeding ground for bacteria that leads to a sinus infection called sinusitis.
- Acute sinusitis may be caused by a viral infection and, therefore, may not respond to antibiotics; it may simply have to run its course. It is, therefore, important to observe acute sinusitis for about seven days prior to initiating an antibiotic therapy. In order to react to allergens, the individual has to be sensitized.
- Food allergy is a fourth condition that may go along with these three atopic diseases.
- It often contributes to the exacerbation of atopic dermatitis, and when that is discovered, elimination of the food in the child's diet helps alleviate the atopic dermatitis symptoms.
- The five most common foods that cause allergies in children are: peanut, soy, milk, egg, and wheat.

WHAT IMMUNE CELLS ARE INVOLVED IN ALLERGIC REACTIONS?

The body has the most effective military system known to Man, called the immune system. The immune system has cells with specialized functions just like in the military.

ACTION OF ANTIGEN PRESENTING CELLS

The process of allergy sensitization starts with exposure of the allergens to an antigen-presenting cell (APC), such as macrophages, monocytes, dendritic cells, or B cells, that I call the "patrolmen" in red at the left bottom corner of the roadmap. These cells live in the skin, the tissues and in the blood.

❖ The patrolmen then present the allergens to the Th0 cell that I call the "white blood cell super-hero or superman," because theTh0 cell can turn into Th2 cells or Th1 cells, depending on the level of danger.

ACTION OF THE TH0 CELL AND B CELLS (BOMB-MAKING CELLS)

❖ The Th0 cell becomes the Th1 cell that is specialized in stimulating B cells (bomb-making specialists) to produce antibodies (smart bombs called IgM and IgG) for fighting bacteria, viruses, protozoa and other non-allergic infectious pathogens.

❖ The Th0 cell becomes the Th2 cell upon exposure to allergens. In the presence of allergens, the patrolmen signal to the superman, which transforms into a Th2 cells that multiplies.

❖ Once the Th2 cells are formed, they produce IL-4 and IL-13 (IL= interleukins, which means between white blood cells, are chemicals used by Th2 cells to communicate — think of these chemicals as the Th2's cell phone or walkie-talkie.

❖ The Th2 cells, in addition to IL-4 and IL-13, also produce IL-5, which generates a late-phase allergy response by stimulating eosinophils (white blood cells specialized in killing parasites), but they also contribute to allergic inflammation by producing toxic proteins (major basic protein, or MBP, and eosinophilic cationic protein, ECP, involved in chronic inflammation and tissue destruction).

❖ The Th2 cells also produce leukotrienes (involved in allergic reactions), IL-3 (stimulates basophils to multiply), and IL-6 (IL-6 is also involved in chronic inflammation).

❖ Th2 cells use the IL-4 and IL-13 chemicals to alert the B cells (bomb-making specialists) that allergens are coming.

❖ The bomb-making cells then make a big bomb called IgE (a smart bomb for fighting allergens).

ROLE OF THE IgE BOMB

❖ The IgE bomb does not explode by itself. It has to find the docking sites.

❖ The B cell is so versatile that it can produce IgE against all allergens (tree, grass, and weed pollens, dust mites, molds, animal dander, cockroach, etc.).

❖ If you view the IgE as a bomb, this bomb does not explode until it attaches to its docking sites, known as IgE receptors.

❖ Once the IgE is formed, it circulates in the blood to find the docking sites.

ROLE OF MAST CELLS (Misery Cell #1) and BASOPHILS (Misery Cell # 2)

❖ The docking sites are on two white blood cells:

- Mast cells (that I call misery cells # 1) live in the skin and tissues

- Basophils (that I call misery cells # 2) circulate in blood vessels with other blood cells.

❖ Once the IgE bomb finds the docking sites, it attaches to them.

❖ At that point, these "Misery Cells," as I call mast cells and basophils because they make millions of people miserable around the world, are armed, dangerous, and waiting for the next encounter to explode.

❖ When an individual is exposed to the same allergen again, the allergen goes through the nose, eventually makes its way to the blood system, and finds the specific IgE bombs made for that particular allergen and that are already on the surface of the misery cells and attaches to them.

❖ The sequence is: bomb attaches to the misery cells then allergens attach to the bombs.

❖ A cross-linking of all the IgE-bomb-allergen complexes occurs on the surface of the misery cells, and that is a signal for these misery cells to explode and pour out their preformed granules in a process called degranulation.

❖ The first chemical granule that is released is histamine.

❖ Histamine is a nerve-ending irritant and causes itching.

❖ That is the reason why you experience the allergy symptoms of itchy eyes, itchy nose, itchy throat, sneezing, runny nose, and, sometimes, itchy skin.

OTHER CHEMICALS RELEASED BY THE MISERY CELLS

❖ If histamine were the only chemical released by mast cells and basophils, the allergy solution would be simple: use antihistamines and there will be no more symptoms. However, the Misery Cells release many more chemicals when they degranulate (a complete list of chemicals released by these cells can be found in the *Allergy Detective: Allergic Rhinitis Treatment Secrets Your Doctor May Not Tell You*).

❖ Two of these chemicals, leukotrienes and prostaglandins, tend to cause late-phase allergic reactions such as: stuffy nose, postnasal drip, coughing, and for asthmatics, constriction of the airways and therefore, wheezing, shortness of breath and chest tightness.

❖ For most patients, the symptoms of stuffy nose, postnasal drip, coughing and other asthma symptoms tend to occur at night because the leukotrienes start coming in the evening and linger through the night.

HOW DO I GET RID OF THE NASAL ALLERGY SYMPTOMS?

To get rid of the allergy symptoms, simply block the chemicals released by the misery cells.

TREATMENT OF HISTAMINE-RELATED SYMPTOMS

❖ To treat the histamine-induced symptoms, antihistamines such as Diphenhydramine (Benadryl®), Loratadine (Claritin®), Desloratadine (Clarinex®), Fexofenadine (Allegra®), Cetirizine (Zyrtec®), and Levocetirizine (Xyzal®) are made and are abundant in the market place.

❖ Zyrtec®, which became available over-the-counter in 2008, is one of the best antihistamines. Allegra®, also very good, is now available over-the-counter.

❖ What I often see in my practice is that patients tend to go for the weakest antihistamines such as Benadryl® and Claritin® first and rarely try Zyrtec® or Allegra® first.

❖ However, though I generally prescribe Zyrtec® or Allegra®, this recommendation may not be optimal for everyone.

❖ I have seen some patients who actually had better results with Claritin® or Benadryl®.

❖ These patients have tried either Zyrtec® or Allegra® and did not get any positive results.

- ❖ Other patients tried Zyrtec®, which led to drowsiness, and therefore they used Claritin®, which is milder and worked better for them.
- ❖ This means that in allergy treatment, one size does not fit all.
- ❖ If you try the more potent antihistamines and you are having problems or you are not getting any relief, try one of the other antihistamines listed above.
- ❖ Individuals, who need to stay awake, such as pilots or air traffic controllers, heavy machine operators and long-distance drivers, should use Allegra® during the day instead of Zyrtec®.

TREATMENT OF LEUKOTRIENES IN ALLERGY SYMPTOMS

- ❖ To block the leukotrienes, montelukast, known as Singulair®, the most popular leukotriene receptor antagonist (LTRA), was conceived, along with other leukotriene receptor antagonists, such as Zafirlukast (Accolate) and others. Children and adults who have allergic rhinitis and asthma symptoms should, therefore, use a combination of a good antihistamine, such as Zyrtec® or Allegra®, and a good LTRA, such as Singulair®.
- ❖ This combination therapy will, in most cases, be optimal.

- ❖ The mistake made by most patients who self-treat and by primary care providers is trying these medications one at a time.
- ❖ Many people first try antihistamines only, and if they do not get good relief, they switch to a LTRA. This stepwise approach to allergy treatment is not effective.
- ❖ Advil Cold and Sinus works to block the prostaglandins, hence Ibuprofen in general can help in some cases.

TREATMENT OF ALL CHEMICALS INVOLVED

- ❖ The master blocker of all these chemicals released by the Misery Cells is a systemic steroid, which is why many health care providers inject steroids or give prednisone to their patients when they present with allergy symptoms.
- ❖ Systemic steroids such as prednisone, however, have multiple undesirable side effects in both adults and children and should be reserved only for short-term bursts for brittle asthma or other severe atopic inflammation.
- ❖ For the treatment of allergic rhinitis, nasal corticosteroids (NCS) that act locally are desirable, and they include:

  Flonase® (fluticasone), which is now generic: approved for ages four and older.

21

Veramyst® (fluticasone): also approved for ages four and older.

Nasonex®: most desirable for children and is approved for ages two and older. Omnaris®, Zetonna® (ceclosenide): approved for ages six and older.

QNasal® (beclomethasone dipropionate): approved for ages twelve and older

Rhinocort AQ® (budesonide): approved for ages six and older, and pregnant women with allergies.

Nasacort AQ® (triamcinolone): approved for ages six and older

❖ Treatment for allergic diseases, therefore, requires a combination therapy: antihistamines to block the histamine released from mast cells and basophils, LTRA to block the leukotrienes, and nasal corticosteroids (NCS) to block all the chemicals that participate in allergic reactions.

TREATMENT OF MULTIPLE CHEMICAL SENSITIVITIES, ALSO KNOWN AS PERENNIAL NON-ALLERGIC RHINITIS (PNAR) or VASOMOTOR RHINITIS

❖ Finally, I explain perennial non-allergic rhinitis (PNAR), often called vasomotor rhinitis or multiple chemical sensitivities.

❖ Eighty-five percent of patients with allergy symptoms also have PNAR.

- ❖ All smokers with allergy symptoms have this condition.
- ❖ Smokers will indicate that cigarette smoke does not bother them. However, once they quit smoking, most smokers cannot tolerate the smell of cigarette smoke.
- ❖ PNAR patients benefit from antihistamine nasal sprays, such as Astelin®, Patanase®, or a combination of Astelin and Fluticasone known as Dymista®.

MEDICATION THERAPY AND TREATMENT TECHNIQUES

- ❖ Once the roadmap is discussed and understood, I then teach the patient how to use the different medications as described below:

START WITH SALINE NASAL SPRAY

- ❖ There are many saline nasal sprays and nasal washes in the market.
- ❖ However, they are not all created equal.
- ❖ If you pay attention to the descriptions of these saline nasal sprays, many report that they compare to Ocean® nasal spray.
- ❖ This means that Ocean® is the standard and all others are mimics.
- ❖ I have tried many of these saline nasal sprays myself and found that Ocean® works better.

❖ I, therefore, recommend that my patients use Ocean® nasal spray not only as a moisturizer for the nose but also for control of postnasal drip.

❖ The persistent, annoying, and often embarrassing postnasal drip that causes most allergy sufferers to clear their throats all the time responds well to Ocean® nasal spray.

❖ However, you have to do it right for good results.

❖ How do you administer Ocean® nasal spray for better results?

❖ I have to call this one Dr. Tano's Technique, my claim to fame.

1. Keep one Ocean® nasal spray bottle in the shower and one with you at all times.

2. While in a hot shower, with nice steam (or on any sink), tilt your head back and gently press the Ocean® nasal spray bottle to let the saline stream into both nostrils, making sure that all the nasal membranes are moisturized. Deliver a generous amount of the nasal spray solution into both nostrils until you get plenty in the throat. Make sure to hold your breath while streaming the solution in the nostrils to avoid gagging. Make sure

the quantity in the throat is large enough to gargle with. Then, cough it up and blow the nose.

Repeat this process five times while in the shower, and clean the nose with water afterward. If you have a stuffy nose, use the nasal spray several times until you can breathe through the nose. Throughout the day, use the spray three times or more for better results.

3. Use Ocean® nasal spray to prevent colds. When you have a sore throat, what do most people tell you to do for relief? Most folks will recommend gargling with hot salt water. Ocean® nasal spray is better than salt water, since it is made isotonic to the secretions from the nose. Using my technique described above, you may prevent getting colds for seven days. As soon as you feel cold symptoms, start using your Ocean® nasal spray as described above. If you are diligent about it, your cold will not last more than two days. I even tell my patients to start using Ocean® nasal spray soon after exposure to someone with a cold or the flu to avoid catching these.

4. Use Ocean® nasal spray to prevent recurrent sinus infections. Sinus infections occur when

mucus accumulates in the sinuses and becomes a breeding ground for bacteria. By draining the sinuses regularly, sinus infections will not occur. If you use Ocean® nasal spray as instructed above, you may be able to drain your sinuses and, hence, avoid recurrent sinus infections. If, after using the nasal spray, you continue to have these symptoms, you should see your allergist for a CT scan of the sinuses for evaluation of chronic sinusitis that may respond to a long-term antibiotic therapy (usually four to six weeks of antibiotic therapy is needed to treat chronic sinusitis effectively). If you start on a long course of antibiotics for your sinusitis, make sure you take good probiotics to prevent a disruption of your intestinal flora. Note that yogurt may not be optimal.

5. Ocean® nasal spray is one of the cheapest ways of treating some allergy symptoms. The 3.5-oz (104 ml) bottle costs about $4 in some stores such as Wal-Mart. If you do not like Wal-Mart, you may find it at Walgreen's or other pharmacies, but it may cost you more. Those of you who follow the adage, "a penny saved is a penny earned," I know where you are heading.

NASAL CORTICOSTEROIDS AND ANTIHISTAMINE NASAL SPRAY TECHNIQUES

❖ The technique for using nasal corticosteroids (NCS's) such as Flonase®, Veramyst®, Nasonex®, Omnaris®, QNasal®, Rhinocort AQ®, or Nasacort®, and antihistamine nasal sprays such as Astelin®, Patanase®, or Dymista® is the same.

Make sure to wait about 10 minutes after using Ocean® nasal spray before using any of the other nasal sprays. If the nose is clean, there will be less sneezing and less runny nose after using the steroid or antihistamine nasal sprays. If you blow the nose after using these medications, you will not get the full benefit. I have noticed that many patients drink their nasal corticosteroids and antihistamine nasal sprays and hope that they get relief from their nasal symptoms. The nose is the problem, and, therefore, the medication should stay in the nose for optimal effectiveness. Even the demonstration insert that comes with these nasal sprays teaches it wrong. The insert says to sniff the spray gently. This is a major mistake because sniffing the spray, takes it directly to the throat and that is what I call drinking the medication. Millions of dollars of nasal spray medications end up in the gut and can even cause sore throat or abdominal upset. The following is the proper technique for these nasal sprays.

❖ To use any of the NCS or antihistamine nasal sprays:
1. Bend the head slightly forward.

2. Insert the nozzle of the bottle into the left nostril as far as possible, slightly
Point the nozzle toward the left eye or if you prefer the left ear, and deliver
two sprays quickly. Lift the head up and pinch the nose gently for the spray to
cover the nasal membranes.

3. Repeat the same process for the right nostril, making sure the nozzle of the bottle points toward the right eye or right ear. (Pointing the nozzle toward the eyes or ear prevents spraying on the nasal septum. Spraying on the septum leads to the nosebleeds experienced by many patients.)

4. I will repeat: Most of all **do not** sniff during the spray or after spraying. Sniffing causes the spray to be lost into the throat and gut. If you sniff your nasal spray, you will be wasting your time and money, and you will not get the expected relief.

NOTE: Astelin®, Patanase or Dymista® (Azalestine + Fluticasone combination) tastes bitter, and if you make a mistake and sniff these during or after the spray in the nose, you will taste these in your throat and mouth. You may wash your throat and mouth with water to relieve the bitterness.

SEQUENCE OF NASAL SPRAYS

If you have concomitant seasonal/perennial allergic rhinitis and PNAR, you may need a combination therapy for better relief from your symptoms.

The most optimal combination is:

1. Ocean® nasal spray
2. Astelin®, or Patinase® or Dymista®
3. Nasal Corticosteroids (NCS)
4. Singulair® (LTRA)
5. Zyrtec® or Xyzal®

❖ Start with Ocean® nasal spray. Wait about 5-10 minutes, and then use the Astelin®, or Patinase® or Dymista®.

❖ Wait another 5-10 minutes and then use the NCS (Veramyst®, Nasonex®, Omnaris®, Qnasal®, Rhinocort AQ®, or Nasacort AQ®).

❖ For most rhinitis sufferers, the adequate amount of Astelin® or NCS is 2 x 2 x 2 (which means two sprays in each nostril twice a day).

- ❖ Most of the time, the 2 x 2 x 1 or the 1 x 2 x 1 recommended by most health care providers does not do the job.
- ❖ Once the acute exacerbation of the rhinitis symptoms improves, use 2 x 2 x 1.
- ❖ In children, use 1 x 2 x 1 if nasal symptoms are mild.
- ❖ For severe nasal symptoms in children, a short course of using the

NCS 2 x 2 x 1 is optimal; then switch to 1 x 2 x 1 when symptoms improve.

- ❖ For the very young (age 1) with severe nasal symptoms, Nasonex®, which is approved for age two and above, can be used off-label (even though not approved for ages below two). In this case, use Nasonex® 1 x 2 x 1.
- ❖ For patients with PNAR, using Flonase®, which has a light floral scent, may not be optimal. Some patients will not tolerate the scent, and they may do better with any of the other NCS's.
- ❖ PNAR sufferers beware! Some insurance plans will refuse to cover other NCS's and direct everyone to Flonase®, which may not be optimal or cost-effective for both patients and insurance companies. In this case, you may want to ask your health care provider to obtain a prior authorization for another brand of NCS.

- ❖ Take the Singulair® around supper time (5:00-6:00 p.m.) because the leukotrienes are released at night, taking the Singulair® in the morning will defeat the purpose. Taking it at bedtime (around 9:00-10:00 p.m. for most people) is too late.
- ❖ Finally, take your Zyrtec® or Xyzal at bedtime. Children six years and older can take Zyrtec® 10 mg or Xyzal 5 mg.
- ❖ By my observation, Zyrtec® syrup does not seem to do the job very well in older children, and many children two-five years old may benefit from using chewable Zyrtec® 5 mg tablets.
- ❖ Nasal allergy symptoms often include eye symptoms (itchy, watery, puffy, red eyes) known as allergic conjunctivitis

TREATMENT OF ALLERGIC CONJUNCTIVITIS
- ❖ For allergic conjunctivitis, you may use an over-the-counter eye drop, such as Zaditor®, or prescription eye drops such as Patanol®, Elestat®, or Pataday®. If you use prescription eye drops, do not expect results immediately. These prescription medications have an antihistamine and a mast cell stabilizer. It takes about two weeks for mast cell stabilization, so be patient.

In addition to these nasal medications and eye drops, I often recommend orthomolecular therapy.

ORTHOMOLECULAR THERAPY

"Orthomolecular medicine, as conceptualized by double-Nobel laureate Linus Pauling, aims to restore the optimum environment of the body by correcting imbalances or deficiencies based on individual biochemistry, using substances natural to the body such as vitamins, minerals, amino acids, trace elements and fatty acids." The term "orthomolecular" was first used by Linus Pauling in a paper he wrote in the journal *Science* in 1968. The key idea in orthomolecular medicine is that genetic factors affect not only the physical characteristics of individuals, but also their biochemical milieu. Biochemical pathways of the body have significant genetic variability, and diseases such as atherosclerosis, cancer, schizophrenia, and depression are associated with specific biochemical abnormalities, which are causal or contributing factors of the illness (definition from www.orthomed.org).

Through anti-aging fellowship training programs, many health care providers are now learning, the principles of orthomolecular medicine to better help their patients.

Biomonitoring, as reported by the CDC, has found harmful chemicals in human blood and urine, and many of these chemicals have been shown by scientific studies to increase estrogen, decrease thyroid function, and decrease androgens (male hormones produced by both men and women). These chemicals are now known as endocrine-disrupting chemicals (EDC's). EDC's not only cause a great deal of the obesity epidemic (and obviously the obesity comorbidities such as diabetes, hypertension, hyperlipidemia, hypothyroidism), but also the growing allergy epidemic (which is estrogen-driven until proven otherwise), and the myriad of other symptoms treated by health care professionals.

How do you protect yourself and your family against pollution and this epidemic of internal chemical disruption? Orthomolecular therapy may contribute to your overall well-being.

ORTHOMOLECULAR APPROACH TO ALLERGIC RHINITIS

I recommend nutritional supplements to enhance the patient's immune system and for overall well-being.

Nutritional supplements I have found useful in an allergy treatment protocol are the following:

- ❖ Nutrient 950 by Pure Encapsulations, a multivitamin that contains NAC (N-acetyl-L-cysteine), all the B-complex vitamins, ascorbic acid, vitamin D3, minerals(calcium, magnesium, zinc, manganese, molybdenum, chromium, and selenium ...), and other nutrients.

❖ EFA Essentials (EPA/DHA, Borage oil). Omega-3 oil also blocks the inflammatory pathway that aspirin and Ibuprofen block and therefore can help alleviate nasal symptoms.

❖ Vitamin D3 helps to alleviate many inflammatory processes, but many people are deficient worldwide. If you live in the Northern Hemisphere, you have a high likelihood of having vitamin D deficiency. The 400 IU RDA is not enough, and many patients need 5000-10,000 IU or more per day to keep their vitamin D level between 50-100 ng/ml deemed to be adequate (normal range 32-100 ng/ml). If you have levels below 50 ng/ml, you should supplement.

❖ Buffered Ascorbic Acid or vitamin C helps to alleviate many inflammatory processes and is also a natural laxative. If you have chronic constipation issues, you may be able to get improvement by using large doses of vitamin C (start with 1000 mg and increase progressively until you have a normal BM and keep taking that dose. If you have diarrhea, it means you have too much) and/or Magnesium. Vitamin C is a good antioxidant and may help to clear free radicals from your body. You are therefore killing several birds out of one stone.

- Co-enzyme Q10 is a big antioxidant that is very useful (sometimes, I recommend a combination of CoQ10 and its reduced form, Ubiquinol)
- The new kid on the block, a big antioxidant, is Astaxanthin. You can try that to help in your free radicals detoxification process.
- Vitamin E (make sure to use mixed tocopherols) is also a big antioxidant
- Aller-Essentials by Pure Encapsulations, which contains quercetin, vitamin C, tinospora cordifolia, hesperidin, methyl chalcone, nettle (urtica dioica), apple polyphenols, beta-glucan (1,3/1,6 glucan), and ubiquinol or CoQ10 is highly recommended for allergies.

Supplementation with antioxidants, such as vitamin C, CoQ10, Astaxanthin, and many other antioxidants has been growing rapidly in the past few years as research on harmful free radicals intensifies. Free radicals are atoms, ions, or molecules with one or more unpaired electrons that bind to and destroy cellular compounds. Dietary antioxidants disarm free radicals through a number of different mechanisms. Foremost, they bind to the free electrons, "pairing up" with them and, creating an innocuous cellular compound that the body can eliminate as waste. Recent research suggests that a synergistic combination of antioxidants is more effective than the total effect of each antioxidant taken alone.

The benefit of antioxidants, minerals, and vitamin D go beyond oxidation and encompass better blood pressure, glucose and lipid controls as well as better control of allergic diseases.

Warning: Nutritional supplements may interact with your other prescribed medications, and you should, therefore, consult with your health care provider prior to embarking on these supplements.

LONG-TERM ALLERGY SYMPTOM RELIEF

All medication treatments for allergies are palliative and will not eliminate the allergy symptoms for a long period of time. To identify the allergens involved in allergic reactions, skin testing and blood testing are performed.

SKIN TESTING AND ALLERGY VACCINE

Two reasons for performing skin testing are:

1.   TIMING OF MEDICATION TREATMENT

- ❖ Spring allergy symptoms are due to tree pollens
- ❖ Summer allergy symptoms are due to grass pollens
- ❖ Fall allergy symptoms are due to weed pollens
- ❖ Year-round (perennial) allergy symptoms are due to cat, dog, dust mites, molds, cockroach, horse, rabbit, guinea pig, hamster, gerbil, mouse, rat, etc.

❖ Patients with spring or fall allergies should pre-empt their season by starting the medication therapy two weeks prior to the beginning of the season, instead of just reacting to the symptoms. Patients with year-round allergies should treat symptoms year-round.

❖ Skin testing is, therefore, performed to guide timing of the medication therapy and for deciding on allergen immunotherapy (AIT), also known as allergy vaccine.

❖ The vaccine takes two forms: subcutaneous immunotherapy, or SCIT, and sublingual immunotherapy, or SLIT.

2.   ALLERGEN IMMUNOTHERAPY

Allergen immunotherapy (AIT), conceived as long-term relief, is designed to specifically restore normal immunity against allergens. The response to AIT is primarily mediated by T-Regulatory cells and B cells. This treatment takes two forms: subcutaneous immunotherapy (SCIT) provided by injection, and sublingual immunotherapy (SLIT) taken orally in liquid form. Both methods stimulate T regulatory cells and B cells equally well and are effective in the treatment of atopic diseases. SLIT is most popular in Europe, but it is making its way into allergy practice in the US. Beneficial effects of allergen-specific immunotherapy include:

- ❖ Decrease in IL-4 and IL-5 production by CD4+ T cells
- ❖ A shift from Th2 cytokine pattern towards increased interferon-γ (IFN-γ) production
- ❖ Rise in allergen-blocking IgG antibodies, particularly of the IgG4 class, which supposedly block allergens- and IgE-facilitated antigen presentation
- ❖ Generation of IgE-modulating CD8+ T cells
- ❖ Reduction in the number of mast cells and eosinophils, including the release of mediators
- ❖ Induction of a tolerant state in peripheral T cells, an essential step in allergen-specific immunotherapy

EFFECTS OF AIT ON T-REGULATORY CELLS AND B CELLS

The response to allergen immunotherapy is primarily mediated by T-Regulatory cells and B cells (think of these two groups of cells as the bomb squad unit; they disarm the bombs). T-Regulatory cells produce IL-10 and TGF-Beta, and B cells produce IgG4 and IgA in the presence of allergen immunotherapy. In response to allergen-specific immunotherapy, the effects of IL-10 and TGF-Beta released by the T-Regulatory cells include:

- ❖ Decreased IgE production by B cells and increased production of IgA and IgG4
- ❖ Decreased IgE-dependent activation of mast cells and basophils
- ❖ Decreased activation and survival of eosinophils

- ❖ Suppressed mucus production by the epithelial cells and reduced airway hyperreactivity
- ❖ Decreased antigen presentation activity of dendritic cells
- ❖ Decreased Th2 cytokine production and suppression of their proliferation

SCIT and SLIT are good, cost-effective and, long-term treatment choices for patients with atopic diseases. However, subcutaneous immunotherapy (SCIT) carries a higher risk of anaphylactic reaction than SLIT.

- ❖ The vaccine, whether SCIT or SLIT, stimulates T-regulatory cells to produce IL-10 and TGF-beta, and also stimulates the B cells to produce IgG4 and IgA instead of IgE.
- ❖ These four "good chemicals" block IL-4 and IL-13 released from the Th2 cells and, therefore, block the communication line between the Th2 cells and the B cells. If the Th2 cells do not communicate with the B cells, then IgE is not released from the B cells. If there is no IgE, then the mast cells and the basophils **generally** do not pour out their chemicals (degranulate). I say generally because the misery cells can degranulate when exposed to other chemicals such as environmental estrogens (more to come on that subject in adult-onset allergies)

❖ These good chemicals also block the mediators released from mast cells and basophils (histamine, leukotrienes, prostaglandins and many more chemicals).

❖ Over time, if the T-Regulatory cells and the B cells are trained long enough to recognize the allergens (it usually takes about three to five years for full recognition). They will do the job on their own, and no allergic reactions will occur for a very long period of time. That is the reason why the allergists recommended the three to five years allergy shots or allergy drops

❖ In the case of SCIT, whether a patient outgrows his allergies or not depends on the strength of the AIT extracts (antigens).

❖ Low-dose therapy is not likely to stimulate the T-Regulatory cells and the B cells to quickly recognize the antigens. The length between allergy injections may also be a problem. If you get monthly injections when you get to your maintenance, your T-Regulatory cells and your B cells are only stimulated once a month and at that frequency, if you are on a low dose allergy injections schedule, you may never outgrow your allergies.

❖ Too high a dose may cause anaphylactic reactions. Hence, SCIT is an art and should be formulated judiciously for an optimal result.

❖ I am of the opinion that patients who are on SCIT should be retested every year to see if they have outgrown any of their allergens, and to reformulate the SCIT protocol to take into account the sensitization pattern at year one, year two, year three, four and five.

❖ By my personal observation, I have seen patients who by year one, have negative skin test to many of their allergens, especially if they are on a high dose injection regimen. I have achieved excellent results by using this method and reformulate the AIT protocol every year. At year five, before discontinuing the AIT injections, skin testing should be performed to ascertain that the patient does not have more allergens that have not been covered.

❖ Sublingual immunotherapy (SLIT) is increasingly becoming popular among US physicians. It is widely used in Europe and recent articles in prestigious American medical journals have indicated that SLIT is as effective as SCIT. Our clinic (Allergy Associates of La Crosse in Wisconsin-website: www.lacrosseallergy.com) is a leading proponent of SLIT in the US and has the longest track record for offering SLIT for environmental allergens and for foods. All our immunotherapy treatment use SLIT instead of SCIT. Sublingual immunotherapy is administered three times daily even if you are at your highest dose. We hold a firm belief that frequency matters. The more you stimulate the T-regulatory and B cells, the more they produce their good chemicals to induce tolerance.

Occasionally, patients have outgrown their allergens by year three or five, but they still have nasal symptoms.

❖ In this situation, chemical sensitivity or estrogens are more often than not the culprits. I will cover the case of estrogen dominance and nasal allergies in the Adult-Onset Allergy Treatment Roadmap. Although the medication therapy (antihistamines, LTRA, nasal corticosteroids) in estrogen-induced mast cell and basophil mediator release is the same as pollen-induced mediator release, these patients may also benefit from bioidentical hormone (hormone with the same structure as the one produced in the body) therapy.

OVERALL SUMMARY

Treatment success of allergic rhinitis is based on the pathophysiology of this disease. When patients come to my clinic, I take a thorough history and perform a physical examination.

After the history and physical examination, I discuss the pathophysiology (The Allergy Treatment Roadmap) of atopic (allergic) diseases as depicted above. The pathophysiology of the atopic diseases diagram shows the interactions between the white blood cells that lead to the release of toxic mediators from the Misery Cells (mast cells and basophils).

I then explain how to block each of these toxic mediators (antihistamines to block histamine, leukotriene receptor antagonists to block leukotrienes, and nasal corticosteroids to block all these mediators). Antihistamine nasal sprays and combination nasal corticosteroid/antihistamine nasal spray are used to treat multiple chemical sensitivities.

Adjuvant therapy with nutritional supplements, vitamins and minerals is also covered. For long-term relief, skin testing is performed to identify the allergens involved. The allergens found determine the seasonality of the allergies and hence clarify the treatment approach. The long-term relief and most cost-effective treatment of allergies involve using allergen immunotherapy. In the US, doctors use two kinds:

subcutaneous immunotherapy (SCIT) and sublingual immunotherapy (SLIT) and both are equally effective.

The vaccine stimulates T-Regulatory cells and B cells to produce four major chemicals that induce tolerance.

This book has tried to answer your questions:

WHY AM I HAVING THE SYMPTOMS?

This question has been addressed by offering the genetic underpinning of allergic rhinitis, Sinusitis, and Conjunctivitis

WHAT IMMUNE CELLS ARE INVOLVED?

This question has been addressed by explaining the working of the immune defense system

- Action of the Antigen Presenting Cells (Patrolmen)
- Action of the Th0-cell (Super-Hero or superman)
- Action of the B-Cells (Bomb-Making Cells)
- Role of the IgE Bomb
- Role of the IgM and IgG Bombs
- Role of Mast Cells (Misery Cell # 1)
- Role of Basophils (Misery Cell # 2)

HOW DO I GET RID OF MY NASAL ALLERGY SYMPTOMS?

This question has been addressed by showing you how you can block the Actual Chemicals Involved (Medication Therapy)

- Block the Histamine
- Block the Leukotrienes
- Block all chemicals involved
- Block multiple chemical sensitivities

And by showing you the medication treatment techniques:

- Saline Nasal Spray-Technique
- Antihistamine Nasal Spray-Technique
- Nasal Corticosteroids-Technique
- Leukotriene Receptor Antagonists-Timing
- Antihistamines-Timing

TO ACHIEVE LONG TERM RELIEF
 Perform Skin Testing and use Allergy vaccine to:
- Determine the timing of medication therapy
- Block the Actions of the Th0-cell (by SCIT or SLIT)
- Block the Action of the Bomb-Making Cells (by SCIT or SLIT)
- Block the Action of Mast cells and basophils (Misery Cells -by SCIT or SLIT)
Determine the effect of Allergen Immunotherapy (AIT)
- Action of the T-Regulatory Cells
- Action of the Bomb-Making Cells

Finally, I want to thank you for purchasing this book. This information has helped many patients and proper use may provide you with good relief from your nasal allergies. This book, however, is not intended to replace your doctor. You should consult with your doctor whenever possible.

If you enjoyed this Nasal Allergy Treatment Roadmap, I would appreciate if you could review this book on Amazon. Your review will help me revise the content and also shape my future treatment roadmap books. If you thought this book was great, please do not hesitate to leave a 5-star review on

Amazon. Watch for other Treatment Roadmaps coming soon.

Enjoy this book and enjoy excellent health.

REFERENCES AND NOTES

For complete references, please visit my website: www.drbtano.com for more information about my other books, *The Allergy Detective: Allergic Rhinitis Treatment Secrets Your Doctor May not Tell You* and *Hormone Imbalance Syndrome: America's Silent Plague-Uncovering the Roots of the Obesity Epidemic and most common diseases*. You may also find these books directly on Amazon at:

www.amazon.com/Hormone-Imbalance-Syndrome-Americas-Silent/dp/0983419205/

www.amazon.com/Hormone-Imbalance-Syndrome-Americas-ebook/dp/B00CLHIEY4/

www.amazon.com/Allergy-Detective-Allergic-Rhinitis-Treatment/dp/0983419221/ and

www.amazon.com/Allergy-Detective-Allergic-Treatments-ebook/dp/B006C2C7CO/

Not all vitamins are created equal and to get your money's worth, you may want to get your professional vitamins on my website or you may buy your vitamins at pure encapsulations website: www.purecapspro.com/toai.

Ortho Molecular, Metagenics and other professional nutritional supplements companies also offer excellent products.

www.ingramcontent.com/pod-product-compliance
Lightning Source LLC
Chambersburg PA
CBHW041221270326
41933CB00001B/3